Angelic-R(... ...

Healing

Level 1

天
恩
SM

Written By
Rev. Debbie Michaels

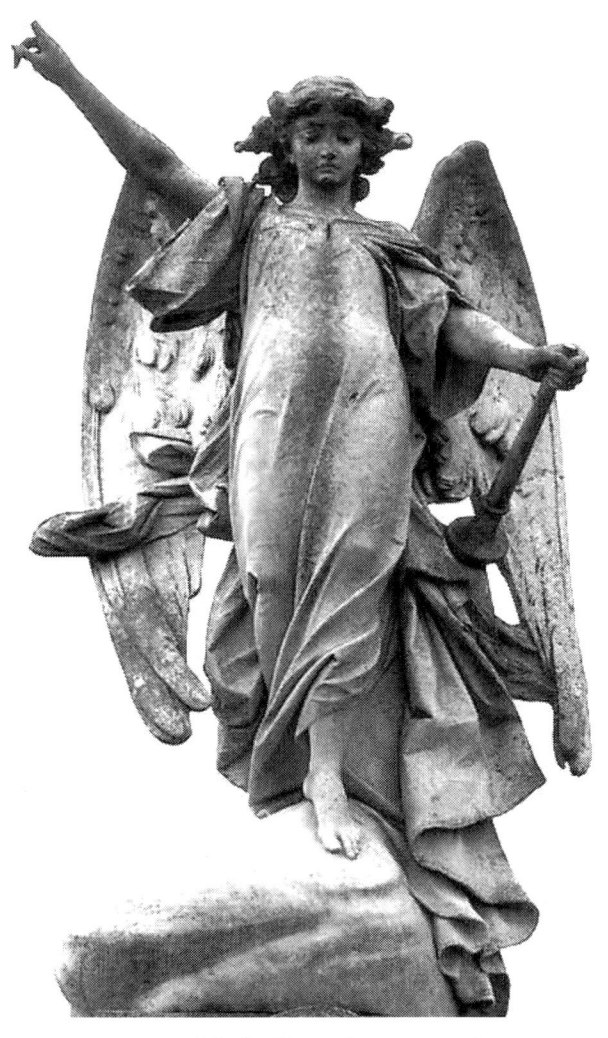

. . . and I shall send you angels
to guard you, to guide you,
and to bless you
Indeed

Attention Future
Angelic-Reiki Energy Healers

Although the Art of Angelic-Reiki Energy Healing is a taught Art, the Angelic-Reiki Healing Energy cannot be taught. Angelic-Reiki Healing Energy is a Gift transferred from Rev. Debbie Michaels God's conduit for Angelic-Reiki Healing Energy, to the Newly Ordained Angelic-Reiki Energy Healing Master.

The Angelic-Reiki Energy Healing Program; is a combination of Angelic-Reiki Attunements and a Sacred Blessing of Angelic-Reiki Healing Energy; This Most Sacred Blessing is preform by Rev. Debbie Michaels.

This Attunement-Blessing May Be Given by Rev. Debbie Michaels, in person or through **Distance Attunement-Blessing**. However, at this time there is no other Human Being who is a Conduit of the *Angelic-Reiki Energy Healing or its 'Ordination Energy.* When the time comes to pass this Sacred Mission on to another Human Being, We the Angels of the Angelic-Reiki Realm will direct Rev. Debbie Michaels to the Being that will take on this Most Holy Mission and all of its responsibilities.

Angelic-Reiki Energy Healing works in harmony with the Human Realm of Traditional Medicine.

Angelic-Reiki Energy Healing is not a substitute for Traditional Medicine, but an addition to it.

We Are Not Medical Doctors.

We Recommend that All Clients Seek Traditional Medical Help by a License Medical Doctor, or Other Health Care Professional; and then abide to their Medical Professional Advise.

Angelic-Reiki Energy Healing
Level 1
Written By
Rev. Debbie Michaels

ACKNOWLEDGEMENTS
This book, as all my books are dedicated to
My Guards and My Guides
The Powers That Be
With My Gratitude
Be Blessed
Indeed

Angelic-Reiki Energy Healing
Level 1
Written By
Rev. Debbie Michaels
Subject to copyright ©

Contact the author at…
www. WhereAngelsGather.org

Angelic-Reiki Energy Healing™
Level 1
Copyright © 2011
Library of Congress Catalog Card Number TX 7-446-439
ISBN 978-1463735883
Where Angels Gather, The Fellowship Inc.

Written By
Rev. Debbie Michaels

Contact the author at...
www.WhereAngelsGather.org

About the Author

After a *Death Experience* on January 2, 2003, Rev. Debbie Michaels began to hear the Angels speak.

Along with her Death Experience came many spiritual gifts. Rev. Debbie Michaels is *The Angelic-Reiki Healing Energy Conduit*, Recognized Clairvoyant, Empath, Spiritual Healer, Ordained Angelic-Reiki Energy Healer Master, Practitioner, Teacher, and Mystic.

In addition to being *The Angelic-Reiki Energy Healing Conduit, Teacher, and Practitioner,* She is also a Usui Reiki Master and Practical Reiki Master.

She became an Ordained Minister on November 11, 2007 and is the founder of...

Where Angels Gather, The Fellowship Inc.

She has also been given *The Gift of Being*, and has channeled the following books, in addition to the one you are about to experience.

Angelic-Reiki Energy Healing
Level 2

Angelic Signs and Symbols
The Language of the Angels

The Art of Angelic Ritual Prayer
Manifesting Miracles

The Art of Angelic Ritual Prayer
Handbook of Divine Energy

The Art of Angelic Ritual Prayer
Book of Divine Herbal Energy

WORDS OF WISDOM:
There Are Things That You May Not Believe In; However, They Are None The Less True.

Table of Contents

Chapter1
Introduction

Angelic-Reiki Healing Energy
Introduction   1-7

Chapter 2
Sanctification Soul, Body and Mind

The Sanctification of the Soul   8-9

Prayer of Purification   10

The Sanctification of
The Mind and the Body with The Soul   11-15

Chapter 3
The Angelic Chakras
Angelic Chakra vs. Standard Chakra   16-17

The purpose of Angelic Chakra Alignment   18-22

Chapter 4
Selecting an Environment and
Preparation
Selecting an Environment   23

Preparation Measures   24-25

Preparing the Client   26-27

Protection and Healing Prayer   28

Chapter 5
Standard Chakras System Balancing

The Standard Chakras System   29-30

Angelic Cleansing and Balancing Prayer   31

The Root/Base Chakra   32-37

The Sacral Chakra   38-40

The Solar Plexus Chakra   41-43

The Heart Chakra   44-46

The Throat Chakra   47-49

The Third Eye/Brow Chakra   50-52

The Crown Chakra   53-57

Energy Balancing Bath or Shower   58-59

Standard Chakra Chart   60-62

Chapter 6
Aura and Aura Clearing

What is an Aura   63-64
Seven Aura Layer   65-68

Aura Interpretations   69-71

Aura Energy Scanning   72

Scanning and Cleansing the Aura   73-74

Reading the Aura   75-76

Angelic-Reiki Aura Clearing   77-80

Chapter 7
Soul Cords and Event Cords vs.
Spiritual Ties and Spiritual Ribbons.

Soul-Cords and Event-Cords vs.   81-82

Spiritual Ties and Spiritual Ribbons   83-84

Chapter 8
Angelic-Reiki Cord Release
Releasing Soul-Cords and Event-Cords

Releasing Soul-Cords and Event-Cords   85-86

*Rele*ase Procedure   87-90

Chapter 9
Angelic-Reiki Healing Meditation
Angelic-Reiki Healing Meditation   91-94

Chapter 10
Wrapping Up   **95**

My Wish for You   **96**

Chapter 1

Introduction
Angelic-Reiki Energy Healing

1

Angelic-Reiki Energy Healing

Introduction:

This as all of Rev. Debbie Michaels books are channeled from the Angelic Realms.

Angelic-Reiki Energy Healing is a gift that was given to **Rev. Debbie Michaels** during her **Death Experience**. Like the Phoenix, she rose again from death, bringing back with her many gifts from our **Divine Creator.**

One of these Gifts is…

…Angelic-Reiki Energy Healing.

And she is now here to share that Gift with you.

Angelic-Reiki Energy Healings are **Spiritual Healing Techniques** that are taught by Rev. Debbie Michaels; in completion of this course, the students receive the Gift of *Angelic-Reiki Healing Energy* through **God's Conduit: Rev. Debbie Michaels.** The students are than transmuted into **Ordained Angelic-Reiki Energy Healing Masters**.

With standard **Reiki Healing Energy**, students are attuned with ancient Japanese Reiki Healing Attunements. However with **Angelic-Reiki**

Energy Healing the students receives not only the *Ancient Reiki Healing Attunements*, but is also infused with *Angelic-Reiki Healing Energy*, through a blessing performed by Rev. Debbie Michaels. This *Angelic-Reiki Healing Energy* is transmuted from the Heavens through Rev. Debbie and is permanently instilled into the newly *Ordained Angelic-Reiki Energy Healing Masters.*

Angelic-Reiki Energy Healing works in harmony with the human realm of *Traditional Medicine.* **It is a Spiritual Healing Practice.**

> **Angelic-Reiki Energy Healing is not a substitute for Traditional Medicine, but an addition to it.**

Angelic-Reiki Energy Healing will *quicken* the healing process by working hand in hand with *Traditional Medicine.* A client should always consult their medical doctor for any and all medical conditions.

Angelic-Reiki Energy Healing **promotes stress reduction and relaxation;** *it also* infuses *Divine Healing Intervention.*

The combination of both these energies creates Miracles.

In Level 1: the practitioner will learn, not only how their *Chakra System* will evolve to a *Angelic Chakra Alignment;* but will also learn the Angelic-Reiki way to balance the ***Standard Chakra System*** of their client, *clear Auras*, and also how *to Release Soul-Cords and Event-Cords*.

Level 2: will introduce the practitioner to the Sacred Symbols of Angelic-Reiki Energy Healing. These Sacred Symbols are extremely powerful keys to Angelic-Reiki Energy Healing. For Angelic-Reiki is an Angelic (Ray Key) of Healing Energy. *A Ray of Divine Healing Energy which is the Key to all Spiritual Healings*.

<u>Notes</u>

4

We are one with God
We are one with the Universe
It is The Divine Truth
That we are
Divinely Entitled
To be
Joyful, Happy,
And
Prosperous
With Divine Intervention
We are blessed
Indeed

Notes

By the Grace of God, Go I

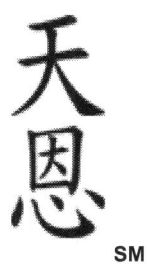
SM

The top symbol represents

GOD

Our Divine Creator

The other symbol represents

GRACE

May the Grace of God find favor in you.

Angelic-Reiki Energy Healing

Angelic-Reiki Energy Healing is Divinely Directed. There are many types of Healing Energies, however, none of which are directly channeled from Our Divine Creator the Supreme Being, *God*, and delivered to us through the *Angelic-Reiki Healing Realm of Angels. It is only channeled by Healers that have been Ordained as Angelic-Reiki Energy Healing Masters* by Rev. Debbie Michaels.

During the ***Ordination Blessing***, *there is a clearing of the Soul, and healing of all its past Karma*. This must be done before the receiving of *Angelic-Reiki Healing Energy*. No other form of energy healing delivers this *Divine Healing Energy*.

Students, who are already Reiki Masters, will receive ***The Angelic-Reiki Healing Energy***, causing an increase in their healing energy, and will strengthen their healing abilities. The vibration that they are accustomed to feeling will become more intense. Their fingers will throb as the *Angelic-Reiki Healing Energy Current* pulses and flows through them and into their client.

Traditional Reiki Masters will be amazed at the difference between the Reiki Energy that they have been using and their ***Angelic-Reiki Energy Healing***.

Angelic-Reiki Healing Energy is the highest form of Spiritual Healing Energy that the *Human Being* is physically capable to control; once again, there is no higher energy.

For this reason, the student must become a *Pure Vessel*; hence, *The Sanctification of The Soul* through *The Clearing of the Soul and The Healing of All Past Karma.*

The student
Will never ever be the same.
The student will be

Healed.

Notes

Chapter 2

Sanctification
Soul, Body and Mind

The Sanctification of the Soul

The Sanctification of the Soul is to make ready the practitioner's soul for the infusion of the Gift of Angelic-Reiki Healing Energy. *We ask that you receive this Gift in a humble, gentle way and with reverence, honoring both Our Divine Creator and The Heavenly Host of Angelic-Reiki Healing Angels.* **You will receive this Sanctification through a Blessing performed by Rev. Debbie Michaels, and also at this time you will also receive the** *Angelic Chakra Alignment.*

The soul is defined by your mind, your will, and your emotions. To become an *Angelic-Reiki Energy Healer,* each of these areas must be purified.

You shall be made *Holy*, for in the acceptance of this *Gift,* you give a pledge to work with the *Angelic-Reiki Realm of Angels, and all of the Healing Light of our Divine Creator.* You shall work with compassion, honesty and love of all *Human Beings*, sharing your *Healing Gifts* to all who are drawn to you.

Thus you will be separate from any other Healers that walk in this world. You shall be *"Holy."*

Notes

You shall be sanctified wholly, *mind, body, emotions, and soul* being kept strong and sound; thus not taking on the illness of the Client during their healing process.

You shall be a consecration in your service. So sanctified in your active assistance as an *Angelic-Reiki Energy Healer*, and totally dedicated to the healing of mankind, a service of love, and compassion.

Notes

<u>Prayer of Purification</u>

Oh Heavenly Angels

Of the Angelic-Reiki Healing Realm

Hear this Prayer of Purification

Make Ready My Soul

Sanctify My Soul

That I May Be Made Worthy

For Your Gift Of

Angelic-Reiki Healing Energy

May I Become a Pure Vessel

Of Your Most

Sacred Healing Energy

Grant Favor Upon My Soul

Grant Favor Upon Me

Notes

The Sanctification of
The Mind, and The Body with The Soul

Our Sacred Soul takes a major role in the Healing of the Body, a balance must be found in the physical world to give peace and honor to this *Our Most Sacred Soul*.

When our soul is at balance, we as *Human Beings* become healthy and happy. We become *Divine Beings of Joy*, our true nature. We make healthy choices, including healthy diets, proper exercise, a true balanced life, including pleasure and love, accepting all of *Divinity's Blessed Gifts*.

When the soul is in balance, it begins to accept the *Healing Energies of the Angeli-Reikic Realm.* Healing all *dis-ease*, neutralizing any and all negative energies. This balance is essential for the maintaining of health and creating an increase for longevity of our human shell.

Joy, love and happiness, are the emotions that carry the highest positive energy frequencies, as *sadness, hate, and loneliness* carry the lowest of frequencies.

As our soul's *rejoices* our human bodies become healthy.

And as our souls *cry*, the body becomes weak.

To live from the *Heart*, is to honor the *Divine Soul;* to laugh, to love, to live life to its' fullest; each moment creates a consciousness of good health, and healing. Thus reducing and destroying toxins that the body may be carrying.

However the soul that is in distress may create an unhealthy life style, causing health problems, causing dis-ease (disease.)

We must develop an awakening for the body to the soul for complete healing.

This is why Angelic-Reiki Energy Healing™ works hand-in-hand with Traditional Medicine.

We honor *both Realms*.

At this very moment, as the knowledge of this course enters your mind, its' *Angelic-Reiki Healing Energy*, begins to infuse you, not only your mind, but also your body, and soul. The entering of this *Sacred Energy* begins your purification. It is of the greatest importance to renew and purify yourself completely, so that your *Sacred Soul* we be able to carry *The Angelic-Reiki Healing Energy*, that you will share with other as *Angelic-Reiki Energy Healers.*

Angelic-Reiki Healing Energy will cleanse the body, naturally, releasing negative energies and emotions that have been stored within us over time and space.

Listed here are several ways that will help purify the soul, the mind, and the body.

- Words have power, and unspoken word have Great Power.

- Say all that is needed to be said.

- Holding our feelings in, good or bad, takes a strain on our soul, causing a weakening to the body, creating dis-ease to the soul.

- Finish what you start in a timely manner, procrastination causes stress.

- Take an inventory of your life, and change what you do not like.

- Eat balance meals, consisting of both meat and vegetables, *Our Divine Creator* provided both for our consumption.

- Cleanliness is next to Godliness; maintain a clean, healthy environment.

- Bathe, in blessed lightly salted water, to ground your energy.

- Quiet yourself daily, be it by sitting quietly, listening to music, or meditating.

- Get at least a minimum of 6 to 8 hours of sleep each day; the human body requires sleep to repair itself.

- Spend time with people and family members that you enjoy. Let go of all other.

- Bring Happiness and Love to each and every opportunity.

- Give thanks to Our Divine Creator, creating "an attitude of gratitude." This creates a whirlwind of positive energy.

- The three L's are very important statues; Live, Laugh, and Love, live by them.

- Desire to Live, engage in a form of creativity.

- Be of Joy, think positive thoughts.

- Smile.

Life is here for us to enjoy, to learn from, to grow with, and to share.

By putting these suggestions into practice we are creating a pure vessel; allowing us to reach our fullest potential.

A vessel worthy of carrying
The Angelic-Reiki Healing Energy.

Notes

Chapter 3

The Angelic Chakras

Angelic Chakra vs. Standard Chakra

What is the difference between the Standard Chakra System and an Angelic Chakra Alignment?

A *Chakra* is the area of interconnection between the body and the soul. Chakras are *wheels of light* which are energy centers in the human body. The chakras are the "gateways of consciousness." It is believe that everybody has seven primary chakras that make up the human energy system.

However with an *Angelic Chakra Alignment,* you receive another *Wheel of Light,* which is an interconnection between *The Human Being* and *Divinity*. You receive *The Divine Chakra.*

The *Angelic Chakra Alignment* also changes the Energy of the Standard Chakras.

Every reflex area in your body will correspond to *The Divine Chakra.* This pure radiant energy spinning at great speeds will strengthen your vibrations, opening you up to a variation of *Divine Healing Energy* from the Angelic-Reiki Healing Realm.

> **Please note:** The Human Being will experience an adjustment period of Forty Day, before The Sanctification of the Soul and Angelic Chakra Alignment is complete.

We recommend the use of the Angelic-Reiki Journal Level 1, 40 Days of Enlightenment, for your journaling. There are (KEY) questions included in the Angelic-Reiki Journal Level 1 to help you during your 40 day adjustment period.

The purpose of *Angelic Chakra Alignment*

The Human Being is made up of energy. Chakras are the vibrations of that energy. Chakras work as a human body's antenna, it receives a wide variety of energetic information that may or may not be used or acknowledged by you. Your body is the electric point through which waves or electric vibrations are able to pass. Every part vibrates with a different frequency of energy. *Angelic Chakra Alignment vibration is at the highest frequency that The Human Being is capable to sustain.*

A Chakras act like a transformer by intercepting energy of similar vibration and links various aspects of the physical body to its non-physical counterparts. *The Human Being* receives information through vibrations and responds to the information to which they are attuned.

Angelic Chakra Alignment will alter and refine that attunement; The Human Being after receiving an Angelic Chakra Alignment, will transform into an ambassador of Divine interceptions and understanding of such information; plus of course The Divine Healing Energy of the Angelic-Reiki Realm.

Angelic Chakra Alignment is given to the Angelic-Reiki Energy Healing student as their first attunement, by Rev. Debbie Michaels, this attunement may be given as a *Distance Attunement, and for those you take the class from other locations including self-home education.*

> Note: An adjustment period of *Forty Days* is required for this Attunement. It is highly recommended that the student keeps a journal, and log down the experiences   that their Physical and Spiritual bodies have during this time.

Angelic Chakra Alignment

8 White   <u>**The Crown**</u>: at the top of the head, *Opens to Receives Angelic-Reiki Healing Energy*

7 Violet   <u>**The Third Eye**</u>: between the eyebrows

6 Blue   <u>**The Throat**</u>: at the back of the neck

5 Green   <u>**The Heart**</u>: at the physical heart

4 Yellow   <u>**The Solar Plexus**</u>: at the abdomen

3 Orange   <u>**The Sacral**</u>: lower abdomen

2 Red   <u>**The Base**</u>: just below the lower abdomen

1 Brown   <u>**The Root**</u>: *Rooted deep into the Physical Realm*

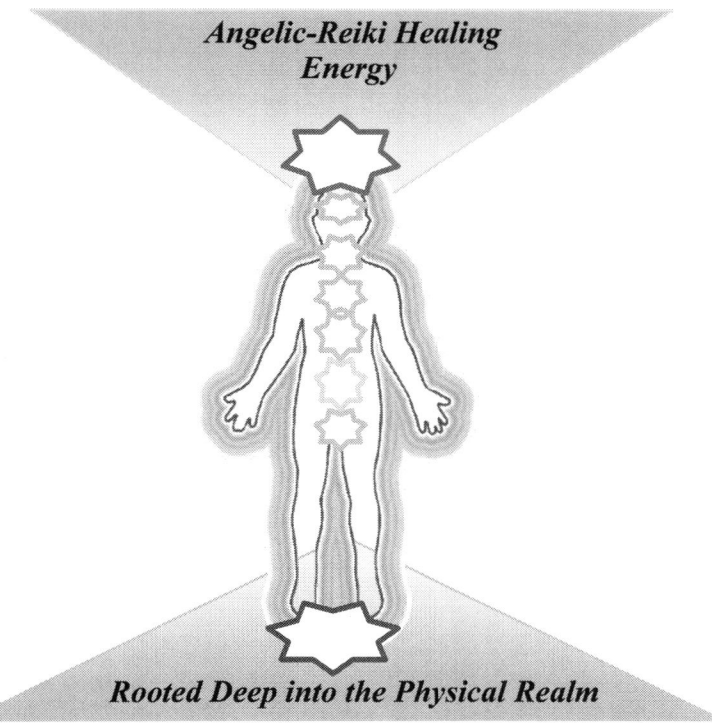

Note: Please remember the first Angelic-Reiki Energy Healing Attunement, is the Sanctification of the Soul and The Angelic Chakra Alignment; and with this attunement is a FORTY DAY adjustment period.

Notes

_____
_____
_____
_____
_____
_____
_____
_____
_____
_____
_____
_____
_____
_____
_____
_____
_____
_____
_____
_____
_____
_____
_____

Chapter 4

Selecting an Environment
And
Preparation

Selecting an Environment

Any and all Angelic-Reiki Energy Healing Treatments may be done out of the practitioner's home, an office, or an alternative medical clinic; as long as it is a location where both the practitioner and client will feel safe and comfortable.

As a practitioner, you may want to set up your own personal Angelic-Reiki Energy Healing Treatment environment to meet your own personal needs. It should be well lit. The location should be a place where you and your client will not be disturbed during *the Angelic-Reiki Energy Healing Session.*

The room should have comfortable chairs and a massage table.

Finally, there should be as little distractions as possible.

Preparation Measures

Just as a surgeon prepares to go into an operating room, so must the Angelic-Reiki Energy Healer prepare.

The practitioner should make sure they are fully energized before beginning an Angelic-Reiki Energy Healing Session. It is recommended to use three sprites of **Angelic-Reiki Energy Healing (A-REH) Charged Holy Water™ to** clear the practitioner's energy field.

Keeping the practitioner's own energy field clear is one of the most important steps to an Angelic-Reiki Energy Healing.

You do not want your energy to become mixed with the client's energy. Once *A-REH Charged Holy Water™* has been spritzed; a protection prayer should be recited. You may use the prayer on page 28. After the protection prayer has been said, the practitioner should once more use three sprites of; *A-REH Charged Holy Water™* this will strengthen their protective barrier.

Remember, *A-REH Charged Holy Water™ is* intended to clear, balance, harmonize, and protect the Practitioner's energy field.

These steps will strengthen the practitioner's well-being and prepare them for the Angelic-Reiki Energy Healing Session.

It is imperative for the practitioner to always protect their own energy field before doing any type of Angelic-Reiki Energy Healing or Spiritual Counseling work.

Energy is free flowing and can affect anyone or anything in its path. When enclosing yourself in the *Angelic-Reiki White Light of Protection*, and the use of *A-REH Charged Holy Water* ™, the practitioner will not take on the emotions or the physical disorders of their clients.

In addition the practitioner should have a small basin of water places in their Healing Room and a clean hand towel. In the basin should be warm water and a table spoon of Angelic-Reiki Energy Healing, Blessed Energy Balancing Salts™ mixed in it.

After each Angelic-Reiki Energy Healing, Procedure the practitioner should rinse and dry their hand to neutralize the energy that they have used during the healing session.

Preparing the Client

After you have set-up the Healing Room, allow
yourself a few moments to relax. Once your client
has arrived, allow the client also to relax after their
drive. The practitioner should then explain what an
Angelic-Reiki Energy Healing is and how it can
help a person translate and address any current
issues that the client may have.

When the client is ready and feels comfortable with
the energy in the room. The practitioner should light
a white candle and welcome *The Angelic-Reiki
Healing Angels* and ask for their assistance, during
this healing session. Envision the flame that is
burning coming from within your soul and reaches
out to connect with *The Angelic-Reiki Healing
Angels,* Also ask for your client's guide(s) to assist
and protect you both during this healing session.

Now have the client either lie down on the massage
table; putting a pillow under their knees, making
them as comfortable and relaxed as possible; or have
the client sit on a chair; where you have the client
lay or sit, depends on the type of healing being
performed.

Once the client is comfortable, the practitioner may
begin the Angelic-Reiki Energy Healing Session.

The *Angelic-Reiki Healing Session* always begins with a prayer of protection and healing.

You will find the Angelic-Reiki Prayer of Protection on the next page and the opening Angelic Healing Prayer on page 31.

<u>Angelic-Reiki Prayer of Protection</u>

Angelic-Reiki Healing Angels,

Ancient Ones and Angelic guides

I ask you to be here at my side

Encompass me and my client please

With the Protective Healing

White Light

Of

Divinity.

Chapter 5

Standard Chakras System Balancing

Standard Chakras System

The chakra system is an arrangement of energy vortexes connecting the layers of the auric field with the major organs and endocrine system of the human body. The chakras directly relate to the amount of energy each chakra absorbs, expels and metabolizes. Hence, if a chakra is blocked the corresponding organ of the physical body will be affected. This *Angelic-Reiki Chakras Balancing* will remove any and all unbalance energy.

The Angelic Chakra Alignment will also enable the practitioner to align and balance their client's *Standard Chakras* with no ill effects.

During the balancing of the Standard Chakras, the client will experience a physical sensation of heat as each Chakra comes into balance. As you work with the Angelic-Reiki Healing Realm to balance each Chakra, the client will become aware of a physical, emotional, and psychological sensation. *The healing of the mind, emotions, body and soul will begin.* The Client may experience tingling, throbbing and warmth during this *Angelic-Reiki Balancing* of their Chakras; it will manifest the nurturing *Energy of Human Life.* The client will also receive *Divine Wisdom* as they come into true balance, this wisdom is from the *Angelic-Reiki Energy Healing; a deeper more profound healing of the mind, the emotions, the body, and the soul.*

Before the *Angelic-Reiki Energy Healing Practitioner* begins to balance their *Client's Chakra System*' an opening prayer to the *Angelic-Reiki Healing Realm* should be performed.

This is easily preformed; by the Angelic-Reiki Energy Healing Practitioner; by reciting a simple yet powerful prayer found on the next page.

Angelic-Reiki Prayer of Healing

I call upon the

Angelic-Reiki Healing Angels

Let your Divine Healing Energy

Enter Me,

Pulsate Through Me

To Cleanse and Balance

The Soul

Of

This

Most Sacred Being

<u>Notes</u>

The Standard Base/Root Chakra

The Standard Base/Root Chakra must be open and functioning before any of your other six chakras will be healed. Therefore, balancing *The Base/Root Chakra* is an important step towards maintaining a healthy chakra system. When *The Base/Root Chakra* is out of balance, physical and psychological ailments may manifest. Those with closed *Base/Root Chakra* are open to autoimmune dis-eases, leg pain, back pain, depression, and insecurity.

As *The Base/Root Chakra is being balanced,* the Client's thoughts should be focused on their ability to manifest a nurturing and secure internal environment so you, the practitioner can begin the balancing of your Client's *Base/Root Chakra.*

Remember: to use **Angelic-Reiki Energy Healing, Charged Holy Water™,** at the beginning of each Angelic-Reiki Energy Healing Chakra Balancing Session; 3 sprits one spritz at the Crown Chakra, the second should be spritzed over the trunk of the client, and the third spritz should be at the foot of the client.

The practitioner begins this balancing by drawing the *Base/Root Chakra* down to the feet of the Client By doing this you **root** *the Base/Root Chakra* deep into the **Physical Realm**, which begin to draw a *taunt energy line* for the balancing of their other six Chakras.

To draw the Root Chakra down to the Client's feet; the practitioner will cup their hands touching their index fingers and thumbs from each hand, thus forming a triangle. They will place their hand approximately six inches above the Root Chakra which is found in the groin area of the Human Being. The practitioner will hold this position until they feel the heat of the Root Chakra, once this heat is felt then, the practitioner will slowly move their hand (still in the triangular position) down to the feet of the Client; holding this position until a throbbing of a heart beat is felt. You are placing the energy field of the **Root Chakra** at the **Base** for your Client. This now becoming (*The Base/Root Chakra*) of the Human Being, adding an excellent grounding point for your Client.

Once the throbbing is felt at the feet of the client, then the practitioner will slowly move back up the client's torso to where the root chakra originates. The practitioner should use their power hand and make three clockwise circles over the chakra, gathering the negative energy. The practitioner's other hand should be palm up in the receiving position. When completed, the practitioner should shake-out their hands to remove the negative energy. Then once again place their hand back over the *Base/Root Chakra*, in the triangular position, and hold till they feel the throbbing of energy in their hands; holding once again till the throbbing feeling begins. At which time **the *Base/Root Chakra*** is balanced. *The Base /Root Chakra* provides the firm foundation necessary to living; establishes personal access to everything needed in order to survive and grow, and offers a basic sense of security and safety.

The Standard Base/Root Chakra's main role is to help *The Human Being* meet basic needs for survival; smoothly, certainly, and with grace. It focuses attention on the daily needs and stimulates the ability to fulfill them.

Note: *The Standard Base/Root Chakra* directs your fight-or-flight responses, feelings of security, and your ability to feel grounded to your present surroundings.

Notes

The Balancing of the Base/Root Chakra

1. The Practitioner should place their hands over the area of the client's lower abdomen; the ***Base/Root Chakra.***

2. Visualize the area between their client's lower abdomen and navel opening up. Imagine the color red flowing from the ***Base/Root Chakra.***

3. The Practitioner should use their mind's eye to make the area glow a beautiful deep red color. When you see this brilliant red color say *"I purify, energize and balance this Sacred Base/Root Chakra."*

4. Take your power hand and make three clockwise circles over the chakra, gathering the negative energy. The practitioner's other hand should be palm up in the receiving position. When completed, the practitioner should shake-out their hands to remove the negative energy. Place your hands back over the ***Base/Root Chakra***, in the triangular position, and hold till you feel the throbbing energy in your hands.

5. Visualize the chakra glowing till it is a brilliant deep red.

6. Visualize the ***Base/Root Chakra*** closing.

7. ***The Base/Root Chakra*** is now balanced.

Notes

Meditation

1 Locate a quiet, peaceful area for performing meditative work. Sit with your back straight and legs uncrossed and feet placed firmly on the floor, with the backs of your hands resting on your lap.

2 Inhale and exhale deeply while clearing your mind. Begin to focus on the base of your spine and visualize an orb of red light forming.

3 Incorporate the ***Base/Root Chakra*** into your meditation your hand postured with palms open to receive healing energy.

4 Chant a combination of affirmations' that will resonate throughout your body to heal and ground the ***Base/Root Chakra***. Chant ***"I am rooted to the Physical Realm and receive its Healing Energy"*** this should be chanted each time you inhale and exhale.

5 Envision earth energy flowing from the ground and up the base of your spine to expand the glowing red orb. Visualize a glowing red light emanating from the orb and expanding to fill the bottom half of your body.

6 See your ***Base/Root Chakra*** spinning in your mind's eye and acknowledge that it is now healthy.

7 End your meditation by affirming, that you are safe, secure, stable and grounded in the ***Physical Realm***.

Notes

_____
_____
_____
_____
_____
_____
_____
_____
_____
_____
_____
_____
_____
_____
_____
_____
_____
_____
_____
_____

The Standard Sacral Chakra

Once the ***Root/Base Chakra*** is properly balanced, the practitioner will begin to move their hands (***still in the triangular position***) up to the ***Sacral Chakra.***

The ***Sacral Chakra,*** or second chakra, and is located in the lower abdomen near the navel and helps us to find balance in our lives. It teaches us to recognize that acceptance and rejection are not the only options in our relationships. The process of making changes in our lives through our personal choices is a product of ***the Sacral Chakra***. It is associated with the colors orange or red-orange.

The Sacral Chakra is an energy center in the body that corresponds physically to the sacrum, in the area located midway between the navel and the base of the spine. ***The Sacral Chakra*** governs bodily fluids, emotions and sexuality.

When ***The Sacral Chakra*** is balanced, you have physical balance and grace; causing feelings of happiness, openness, trust, and the ability to turn problems into a challenges.

Keeping Your Sacral Chakra in Balance

Sit in a comfortable position and center yourself. Picture a beam of healing energy flowing down your head and through your body. Next picture energy being pulled up from the earth, and spreading throughout your body. When you feel the calm flow of energy, proceed to the next step.

Visualize the *Sacral Chakra* with a beam of orange light entering your body growing larger and stronger. As you exhale, picture the energy radiating throughout your whole *Sacral Chakra*. Keep this focus until you feel the sensation of heat. Once you experience this sensation of heat, you have restored the energy to the *Sacral Chakra.*

The Balancing of The Sacral Chakra

1. The Practitioner should place their hands over the area of the client's lower abdomen; (the practitioner's hands should still be in the triangular position) let your hands hover there.

2. Visualize the area between your lower abdomen and navel opening up. Imagine the color orange flowing from the *Sacral Chakra*.

3. The Practitioner should use their mind's eye to make the area glow a beautiful deep orange color. When you see this brilliant orange color, say *"I purify, energize and balance this Sacred Sacral Chakra."*

4. Take your power hand and make three clockwise circles over the chakra, gathering the negative energy. The practitioner's other hand should be palm up in the receiving position. When completed, the practitioner should shake-out their hands to remove negative energy. Place your hand back over the *Sacral Chakra*, in the triangular position, and hold till you feel the throbbing energy in your hands.

5. Visualize the chakra glowing till it is a brilliant deep orange.

6. Visualize the *Sacral Chakra* closing.

7. *The Sacral Chakra* is now balanced.

<u>Notes</u>

The Satandard Solar Plexus Chakra

The Solar Plexus Chakra, or third chakra, is located at the abdomen *The Solar Plexus Chakra* is described as a vital network of nerves. It emanates from the abdomen and connects various nerves that branch out into the body; and it also connects to various organs, such as the stomach, spleen, liver, pancreas and esophagus. In short, *The Solar Plexus Chakra* is a very delicate and complex cluster of nerves that acts as a connection to many important organs of the nervous and digestive systems.

The Solar Plexus Chakra is also linked to our emotions, which reacts to thoughts of worry, anxiety, excitement, or fear. Located just above the navel, the balance of *The Solar Plexus Chakra* affects the integrity of our skin, digestive organs, stomach, pancreas, liver and endocrine glands.

The Solar Plexus Chakra located in your solar plexus, halfway between the navel and ribcage-is the domain of intellect. It is the center of *The Human Being's* intellect and personal power, giving them the ability to stay true to their course in life. Courage, integrity, and choice, are the backbone of this sphere. It rules your self-direction, self-control, personal will and physical energy.

A well-balanced *Solar Plexus Chakra* results in high self-esteem and the ability to accept responsibility for human life.

The Balancing of the Solar Plexus Chakra

1. The Practitioner should place their hands (the practitioner's hands should still be in the triangular position) over the area of the client's upper abdomen; let your hands hover there.

2. Visualize the area between your upper abdomen and rib-cage opening up. Imagine the color yellow flowing from the *The Solar Plexus Chakra*.

3. The Practitioner should use their mind's eye to make the area glow a beautiful bright yellow color. When you see this brilliant yellow color, say *"I purify, energize and balance this Sacred Solar Plexus Chakra.*

4. Take your power hand and make three clockwise circles over the chakra, gathering the negative energy. The practitioner's other hand should be palm up in the receiving position. When completed, the practitioner should shake-out their hands to remove negative energy.

5. Place your hand back over *The Solar Plexus Chakra* in the triangular position, and hold till you feel the throbbing energy in your hands.

6. Visualize the chakra glowing till it is a brilliant yellow.

7. Visualize *The Solar Plexus Chakra* closing.

8. *The Solar Plexus Chakra* is now balanced.

Notes

The Standard Heart Chakra

The Heart Chakra also referred to as the fourth chakra; is located exactly where your Heart is located, in the center of your chest. *The Heart Chakra* carries both male and female energies. It controls your emotions, compassion, love and general well-being.

An inadequate or excessive energy flowing through *The Heart Chakra* may cause problems, such as being over- emotional or under-emotional, uncompassionate and unloving.

It is extremely important to keep *The Heart Chakra,* in balance for our general well-being and the evolution of our Soul. The balancing of *The Heart Chakra* keeps us connected to the Divine Energy.

Located near your heart, in the very center of the chest, *The Heart Chakra* is the sphere of human intimacy. It is affects our feels of warmth, nurturing, friendship and family. *The Heart Chakra* is the seat of *The Human Being's* ability to feel joy, unity, laughter and especially, love; the very highest power in *The Human Being's* life. It expands *The Human Being's* capacity to be generous, sensitive, forgiving and tolerant.

With a balanced *Heart Chakra*, the circulation of *The Human Being's* blood is healthy and smooth, the heart rhythm is regular and the arteries are clear from blockage.

The Balancing of the Heart Chakra

1. The Practitioner should place their hands over the area of the client's heart; (the practitioner's hands should be in the triangular position) letting their hands hover there.

2. Visualize the area between the rib-cage, opening up. Imagine the color green flowing from the *Heart Chakra*.

3. The Practitioner should use their mind's eye to make the area glow a beautiful brilliant green color. When you see this brilliant green color, say *"I purify, energize and balance this Sacred Heart Chakra."*

4. Take your power hand and make three clockwise circles over the chakra, gathering the negative energy. The practitioner's other hand should be palm up in the receiving position. When completed, the practitioner

should shake-out their hands to remove negative energy. Place your hand back over the *Heart Chakra*, in the triangular position, and hold till you feel the throbbing energy in your hands.

5. Visualize the chakra glowing till it is a brilliant green.

6. Visualize the *Heart Chakra* closing.

7. *The Heart Chakra* is now balanced.

Notes

The Standard Throat Chakra

The Throat Chakra is the fifth energy center and is located at the back of the neck. On an energy level, it is the center of personal expression and the messenger of the soul.

The throat chakra is located where food, drink, drugs, smoke and other external substances enter your body. That's why it is extremely important that *The Human Being* makes a conscious choice to ingest healthy, wholesome substances instead of those that can harm the body and the soul.

In the *Human Being's* body *The Throat Chakra* governs throat, thyroid, trachea, esophagus, neck, mouth, teeth, and ears.

The Throat Chakra rules your communication, and creativity. *The Throat Chakra* awakens *Human Beings* to the truth that life is built on words, thoughts, beliefs and ideas.

A well-balanced *Throat Chakra* enables the ability of speaking and listening, it also governs creativity and awakens the ability to connect with others. *The Throat Chakra* also tunes into the inner voice, allowing *The Human Being* to connect with *The Almighty Creator.*

To keep *The Throat Chakra* balanced the expression of needs and establishing boundaries are extremely important. Speaking the truth of the Soul can be difficult. Especially when trying to convey anger. Please remember that there is nothing inappropriate about having feelings and expressing them when they stand up for truth and justice.

The Balancing of the Throat Chakra

1. The Practitioner should place their hands over the area of the client's throat; (the practitioner's hands should be in the triangular position) letting their hands hover there.

2. Visualize the throat area opening up. Imagine the color light blue flowing from the *Throat Chakra*.

3. The Practitioner should use their mind's eye to make the area glow a bright light blue color. When you see this bright light blue color, say "*I purify, energize and balance this Sacred Throat Chakra.*"

4. Take your power hand and make three clockwise circles over the chakra, gathering the negative energy. The practitioner's other

hand should be palm up in the receiving position. When completed, the practitioner should shake-out their hands to remove negative energy. Place your hand back over the **Throat Chakra**, in the triangular position, and hold till you feel the throbbing energy in your hands.

5. Visualize the chakra glowing till it is a bright light blue.

6. Visualize the **Throat Chakra** closing.

7. **The Throat Chakra** is now balanced.

Notes

The Standard Third Eye/Brow Chakra

The *Third Eye/Brow Chakra* is the link between *The Human Being's* highest consciousness and basic instincts. Located between the eyes, this chakra influences the integrity of our brain, eyes, ears, nose, nervous system and pituitary gland.

The Third Eye/Brow Chakra is associated with the color indigo blue, the sixth chakra is located between and just above the physical eyes, creating the spiritual *Third Eye* While our two eyes see the *Physical World*, our sixth chakra sees beyond the physical. This vision includes clairvoyance, telepathy, intuition, dreaming, imagination, and visualization.

The *Third Eye/Brow Chakra* will involve *The Human Be*ing in both the creation and perception of art, and has a powerful impact on *The Human Being*; even when they are not aware of it. *The Human Being* is sensitive to the images found in everyday life.

A balanced *Third Eye/Brow Chakra* leads to Self-evaluation, truth, intellectual abilities, feelings of adequacy, and openness to ideas of others, ability to learn from experiences, emotional intelligence, clairvoyance, intuition and insight.

When the *Third Eye/Brow Chakra* is excessively active with energy, headaches, hallucinations, nightmares, and difficulty concentrating can be experienced.

When the *Third Eye/Brow Chakra* is deficient, we have a poor memory, experience eye problems, have difficulty recognizing patterns, and can't visualize well. Keeping the *Third Eye/Brow Chakra* in balance is necessary for the Human Being. Also, creating positive images and visualizations is a practice that helps improve and creates a healthy *Third Eye/Brow Chakra*.

The Balancing of Third Eye/Brow Chakra

1. The Practitioner should place their hands over the area of the client's forehead; (the practitioner's hands should be in the triangular position) letting their hands hover there.

2. Visualize the forehead area opening up. Imagine the color of indigo blue flowing from the *Third Eye/Brow Chakra*.

3. The Practitioner should use their mind's eye to make the area glow a bright indigo color.

When you see this bright indigo blue color, say *"I purify, energize and balance this Sacred Third Eye/Brow Chakra."*

4. Take your power hand and make three clockwise circles over the chakra, gathering the negative energy. The practitioner's other hand should be palm up in the receiving position. When completed, the practitioner should shake-out their hands to remove negative energy Place your hand back over the *Third Eye/Brow Chakra*, in the triangular position, and hold till you feel the throbbing energy in your hands.

5. Visualize the chakra glowing till it is a bright indigo blue.

6. Visualize the *Third Eye/Brow Chakra* closing.

7. *The Third Eye/Brow Chakra* is now balanced.

Notes

The Standard Crown Chakra

The Crown Chakra representing the flow of energy in *The Human Being's* body and soul; it is located at the top of the head to receive energies from above. *The Crown Chakra* is associated with the sixth sense and living in the present.

The Crown Chakra is an energy link to the nervous system, brain and pineal gland. The function of *The Crown Chakra* is thought, and this chakra is associated with *The Human Being's* highest functions of its mind. Even though the mind cannot be seen nor felt, it creates the belief systems that control our thoughts and actions.

The Crown Chakra symbolizes the highest state of enlightenment and enables *The Human Being's* spiritual development. The seventh chakra is like a violet halo on the top of the head.

The Crown Chakra is filled with so many thoughts it is necessary to keep it in balance. By keeping *The Crown Chakra* in balance, it is opened to experience the Divine, to be opened to a higher and deeper understanding of Divinity. Meditation, allows the mind to become more present, clear, and insightful. It is a quieting of the mind that allows *The Human Being* to experience Divinity.

The Crown Chakra is the connection for *The Human Being's* ability to trust something more powerful than themselves, to trust in *The Almighty Creator* and *The Angels.*

The Human Being's values, ethics, courage, selflessness, the ability to see a larger purpose, faith and inspiration, enters *The Human Being's* through *The Crown Chakra.*

The Balancing of the Crown Chakra

1. The Practitioner should place their hands over the area of the client's head; (the practitioner's hands should be in the triangular position) letting their hands hover there.

2. Visualize the head area opening up. Imagine the color of a brilliant violet flowing from the *Crown Chakra.*

3. The Practitioner should use their mind's eye to make the area glow a brilliant violet color. When you see this bright violet color, say *"I purify, energize and balance this Sacred Crown Chakra."*

4. Take your power hand and make three clockwise circles over the chakra, gathering the negative energy. The practitioner's other hand should be palm up in the receiving position. When completed, the practitioner should shake-out their hands to remove negative energy Place your hand back over *The Crown Chakra*, in the triangular position, and hold till you feel the throbbing energy in your hands.

5. Visualize the chakra glowing till it is a brilliant violet.

6. Visualize *the Crown Chakra* closing.

7. *The Crown Chakra* is now balanced.

Remember: at the end of the Chakra Balancing Sessions to use **Angelic-Reiki Energy Healing, Charged Holy Water™, this** seals the balancing process; one spritz at the Crown Chakra, the second should be spritzed over the trunk of the client, and the third spritz should be at the foot of the client.

To help keep the **Chakra System in Balance** it is recommended to use three spritzes of **Angelic-Reiki Energy Charged Holy Water ™** at the end of each day, or as needed.
Spray three sprites over the Crown Chakra.

Meditation

1 Locate a quiet, peaceful area for performing meditative work. Sit with your back straight and legs uncrossed and feet placed firmly on the floor, with the backs of your hands resting on your lap.

2 Inhale and exhale deeply and clear your mind. Begin to focus on the top of your head and visualize an orb of violet light forming.

3 Merge *The Crown Chakra* into your meditation; your hand postured with palms open to receive healing energy.

4 Chant a combination of affirmations that will resonate throughout your body to heal and ground *The Crown Chakra*. Chant "l am rooted in the *Physical Realm and now opened to the Spiritual Realm ready to receive the Angelic-Reiki Realm's Healing Energy*" should be chanted each time you inhale and exhale.

5 Envision Divine energy flowing from the Heavens into your mind, body, and soul expanding and glowing a bright violet.

6 See *The Crown Chakra* spinning in your mind's eye and acknowledge that it is now healthy.

7 End your meditation by affirming, that you are safe, secure, stable and grounded in the *Physical Realm.*

Remember the practitioner should have a small basin of water places in their Healing Room and a clean hand towel. In the basin should be warm water and a table spoon of Angelic-Reiki Energy Healing, Blessed Energy Balancing Salts™ mixed in it.

After each Angelic-Reiki Energy Healing, Procedure the practitioner should rinse and dry their hand to neutralize the energy that they have used during the healing session.

Notes

Energy Balancing Bath or Shower

After Balancing Chakra and working with the Energies, the practitioner may want to take a bath or shower to help Balance their own energy, and bring it down to a more *Human Frequency*. Working with Energy can either drain a person or highly energies a person; In the case of Balancing Chakras, the practitioner will be *Highly Energized*. When working with the Angelic-Reiki Realm, the practitioner raises their vibration.

On this page and the next page, I have included a couple of ways to bring the *Practitioner* back down to their normal human frequency.

An Energy Balancing Bath

Rehydrate your body. Water calms, energizes, relaxes and strengthens the body. Soaking and drinking water are all good ways to accomplish this. Drinking 2 liters of water daily will ensure that your body is flushing toxins and waste.
Meditate in water. Fill your tub with warm water. Add bath salts and essential oils such as rose, gardenia or sandalwood to the bath water; you may also choose to use **Angelic-Reiki Energy Healing, Energy Balancing Bath Salts™** Dim the lights and relax in the tub and meditate on your Chakras being in perfect balance, for at least 20 minutes.

Also you may burn incense to take advantage of aromatherapy. Certain scents will help balance the chakras. To balance the chakras, incense should have a particular scent, such as gardenia, sandalwood, ylang-ylang, patchouli, rose, or amber.

An Energy Balancing Body Wash for Showering

To balance the chakra, mix sea- salt in flakes with olive oil or sesame oil in a ratio of one handful of salt to one tablespoon of oil. Form a paste. A drop of rose or lavender essential oil can also be added to the mixture. Or you may also use **Angelic-Reiki Energy Healing, Energy Balancing Body Wash™**

Stand in a warm shower for a minute or two, step away from the water and massage the salt mixture into your body, starting at the feet, using circular movements in a clockwise direction with the whole hand. Work your way up to the legs, the abdomen, back and the chest.

Move to the hands and work up the arms to the shoulders, moving toward the direction of your heart. Rinse under the warm water.

Standard Chakra Chart

Chakra	Color	Focus Point
1 Root Chakra Located at the base of the spine	**Red**	Stability, grounding, security, physical energy, will
2 Sacral Chakra Located below the navel	**Orange**	Creativity, sexuality reproduction, and desire, emotion
3 Solar Plexus Chakra Located at solar plexus	**Yellow**	Intellect, ambition, personal power
4 Heart Chakra Located at center of the chest	**Green**	Love, compassion, emotional balance

Chakra	Color	Focus Point
5 Throat Chakra Located at the neck	**Blue**	Communication, expression, divine guidance
6 Third Eye Chakra Located center of forehead	**Indigo**	Spiritual awareness, intuition
7 Crown Chakra Located at the top of the head	**Violet**	Enlightenment, cosmic consciousness, energy, perfection.

Standard Chakras Alignment

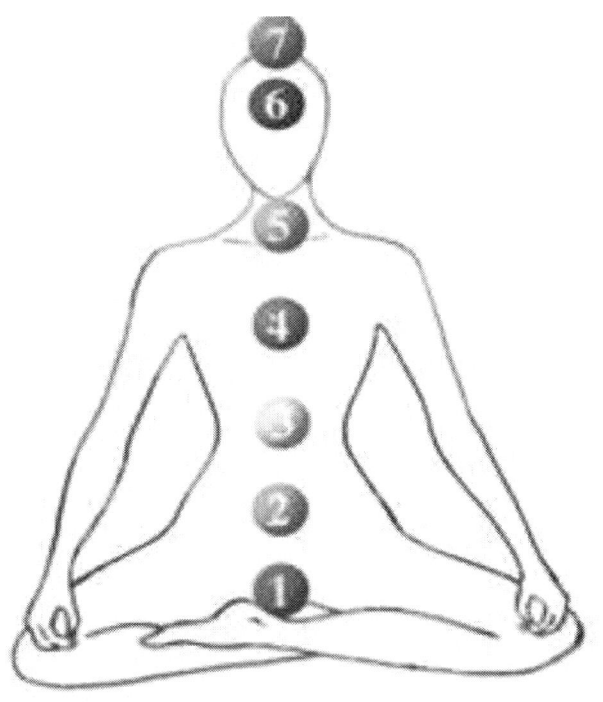

Notes

Notes

Notes

Chapter 5

Aura and Aura Clearing

What is an Aura?

An *Aura* is a field of subtle energy, surrounding a person or object. The *Aura* is partly composed from electromagnetic radiation both low and high frequencies.

Low frequency such as human body heat is related to the lower levels of the functioning body; whereas high frequency associated with our conscious activity such as thinking, creativity, intentions, sense of spirituality.

These energies are drawn from both the *Heavens* and *Earth* Every living thing on the earth radiates a field of energy, which is called an *Aura*. In the *Human Being*, there are seven main centers in the body that produce the energy of the aura, as you know these energy centers are the *Chakras*.

Notes

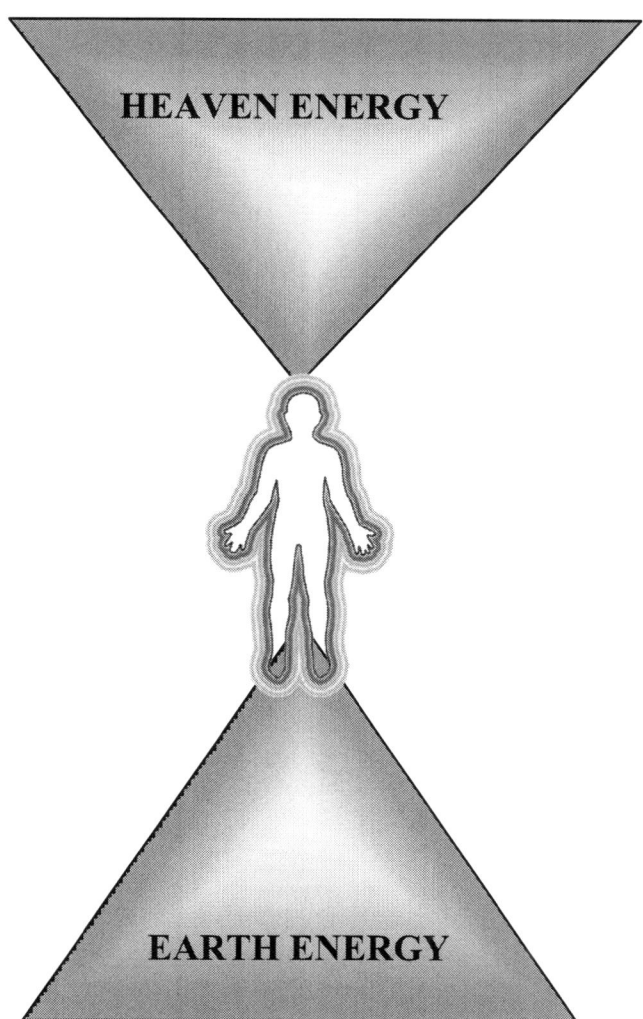

Notes

Seven Aura Layers:

The formation of the seven layers, along with the shape, depth and assembly of colors of the *Aur*a, make it so obvious, spiritual and yet earthly, that it becomes a very useful tool for the study of the *Human Being.*

The Etheric Body Layer:

Etheric Body layer: It depicts the physical condition. It forms a bright circle around a healthy person, while it is a pale appearance around an ailing person.

Etheric Body Layer: Physical sensation

Consciousness layer: Consciousness is the sensations such as physical pleasure or pain. Expression of Health: Natural metabolism of energy, which maintains structure and function of etheric body.

Chakra: 1st Base/Root

Color: Red

Emotional Layer

Emotional layer: Depicts the status of emotions.

Consciousness layer: Expresses basic emotions and reactions like fear, anger and love.

Chakra: 2nd Sacral

Color: Orange

Mental Layer:

Mental layer: It reflects the internal energy of a person and indicates the will power.

Consciousness layer: Expression of Consciousness: Thinking expressed in terms of rational thinking.

Chakra: 3rd Solar Plexus

Color: Yellow

The "Astral" Body:

Astral layer: The central astral layer is connected with the heart, provides a link between body, mind and soul and connects the individual with other living beings in the universe. It is big and bright in those who value relationships with others.

Consciousness Layer: The "Astral" Body: "I love humanity"

Chakra: 4th Heart

Color: Green

The Etheric Temple Layer:

Etheric Temple layer: The energy field of communication and creative expression. Blockage, black-brown spots, clouds or darkness in this layer indicate the feeling of isolation.

Consciousness Layer: Higher Will the act of willing things into existence, Divine Will: "Thy will and mine are one."

Chakra: 5th Throat

Color: Light Blue

The Celestial Body:

Celestial layer: Represents the visual senses. It also reflects an individual's outlook about the rest of the world.

Consciousness Layer: Higher Feelings expresses itself as higher feelings like universal love; love that goes beyond human beings and friends into a universal love for all life.

Chakra: 6th Third Eye

Color: Indigo Blue

The Ketheric Layer:

Ketheric layer: Linked with self-confidence & decision making ability. When it is shining brightly, it indicates a mind unafraid of judgments and criticism by others.

Consciousness layer: Consciousness is expressed in higher concepts of knowing or belief systems. This is where the initial creative impulse begins; not just linear knowing, but integrated knowing."

Chakra: 7th Crown

Color: Golden

Angelic-Reiki Aura Color

Aura Interpretations

There are *6 facets* to perceiving and interpreting the layered energy of an aura. Layers are determined by *color, variations, the shapes, consistencies, clarity and the vibration.*

Most methods of aura reading define particular meanings for each color in the spectrum. For Angelic-Reiki Energy Healing, the list below is used for reading and scanning the aura.

BLACK: Often seen around abused children, divorces, drug addicts and torture victims.

GREEN: Friendly people

ORANGE: Strong motivation

YELLOW: Inspiration

BROWN: Indicates a person with common sense

RED: Short tempered

BLUE: People with this color tend to move slow, but safe and sure

INDIGO: Strong psychic ability

VIOLET: Once again humble people

GOLD: A higher level of consciousness

Become familiar with these *common interpretations* of the primary colors form. You then should be able to interpret the more complex colors of the spectrum; these combinations of colors generally take on the combined meaning of the primary colors.

The clarity or brightness of the color also plays a key role in color interpretation. Very often a color that appears cloudy has the opposite meaning of its vibrant and clear counterpart. A vibrant red means the subject has anger issues to work out. A dull or cloudy red indicates frustration.

As you learn color definition, you should also become familiar with the location of the color and how the two relate. The location, consistency and clarity of a color within the aura help to determine their full meaning. A vibrant yellow around the chest area indicates love, sympathy, and tolerance.

You may see a color localized in a specific area. But if you look at the entire aura overall, regardless of layers or color, you may see a hole in the aura. This could indicate a dysfunction in the human body, such as a dis-ease or injury.

Notes

Aura Energy Scanning

Scanning, and then interpreting the analysis of the aura will give the practitioner an evaluation of the spiritual status of their client.

The Aura provides a much more complete picture in regards to the state of *Being*. It indicates the relationship of harmony, success, obstacles, physical health and emotional health.

Also, sometimes a chakra may shut down due to blocks in the energy field and stops emitting the energy. This may be caused due to trauma, illness, or some other imbalance; whether it is physical, emotional, mental or spiritual.

An analysis is very significant and if required, an Angelic-Reiki Energy Healing Aura and Chakra cleansing is advised.

Notes

Scanning and Cleansing the Aura
Aura Scanning

The practitioner will be doing this *Angelic-Reiki Aura Scanning* with the awareness that they will be receiving, information on the energy field of the client. Begin healing session by reciting clearing prayer on page 31.

The concentration on the body outline will probably require a little effort, at least while learning and being confident in scanning the *Aura*.

Remember: to use **Angelic-Reiki Energy Healing Aura Clearing Holy Water™** at the beginning of each **Angelic-Reiki Energy Healing Aura Clearing Session** one spritz at the Crown Chakra, the second should be spritzed over the trunk of the client, and the third spritz should be at the foot of the client

---

Before beginning treatment, stand with your eyes closed and invite the *Angelic-Reiki Angels* to assist you in your preparation for the client's scan. Ask that both you and your client be engulfed with the **White Light** of *Their Angelic-Reiki Protection*. Release all effort, and open yourself up to the effortless reception of *Their* angelic information.

Let go of all personal thoughts and preconceptions, suspend your thinking.

The information will appear as patterns of blotches or patterns of spots on the body, fuzzy areas, or other appearances in the aura's colors.

The Practitioner with be seeing information intuitively with the *third eye chakra*. Each person will perceive this information differently.

You must experience, and interpret it for yourself; to understand your own unique perceptions.

The practitioner will sense many conditions in the client, and in various combinations, depending on the client's condition. The practitioner may, at the same time, receive information regarding the proper treatment for these areas the practitioner will not be limited, in their reading, to "intuitive sight," as information may come also through "sounds" or "feelings."

When the practitioner is receiving clear Angelic-Reiki information they are free from thoughts and emotions, free from the excessive activity of the "thinking mind." This information coming from the Angelic-Reiki Realm has a wider awareness. The practitioner must learn for themself how this difference feels.

Reading the Aura

The practitioner will be doing this with the mindfulness that they will be receiving, information on the energy field from the *Angelic-Reiki Healing Angels*. The focusing on the client's body outline will probably require a little self-discipline, at least while learning.

Before beginning treatment, stand with your eyes closed and concentrate, imagine in your third eye views the shape of your client's body, and then the body outline.

Release all effort, and open yourself up to the reception of the information that will come. Let go of all thoughts and presumptions. The Practitioner will know intuitively, with the third eye chakra the well-being of its client. Each person will receives information differently. You must experience, and interpret for yourself, your own unique perceptions.

The practitioner will sense many conditions in your client, in various combinations, depending on the client's unique condition. The practitioner may also, receive information regarding the proper treatment for these areas. The practitioner will not be limited, in your reading, to "intuitive sight," as information may come also through the other senses, such as sound or feelings.

When the practitioner is receiving clear Angelic-Reiki information they are free from thoughts and emotions, free from the excessive activity of the "thinking mind.

This information coming from the *Angelic-Reiki Realm* and has a wider awareness. The practitioner must learn for themself how this difference feels.

Remember the practitioner should have a small basin of water places in their Healing Room and a clean hand towel. In the basin should be warm water and a table spoon of Angelic-Reiki Energy Healing, Blessed Energy Balancing Salts™ mixed in it.

After each Angelic-Reiki Energy Healing, Procedure the practitioner should rinse and dry their hand to neutralize the energy that they have used during the healing session.

Angelic-Reiki Aura Clearing

It is vital to the health of the client that the flow of energy is free from any obstacle; from any stagnant, and unhealthy contaminated energies that can block its normal flow. If you have detected such energies in the aura of your patient, they may be cleared out and removed by using a procedure known as *Angelic-Reiki Aura Clearing.*

This technique is performed over the various areas of the body where this energy occur, as well as over chakras uses the practitioner's hands to remove undesirable energies from the lower layers of the energy field.

While performing aura clearing, the hands are moved in a particular fashion. The practitioner will "draw out" and away from the body of the client, removing the auric energy toxins. This movement is done in a slow, deliberate manner the practitioner must concentrate on the act during *Angelic-Reiki Aura Clearing*.

The practitioner should place their power-hand palm-down over the crown chakra (at this time you should invoke the *Angelic-Reiki Healing Angels* to direct them in the Clearing and Cleansing of the Client's Aura. With their fingers spread wide begin passing your hand slowly down the frame of your client. Your fingers should extend straight out, level from the hand. The hand, at the beginning of the drawing motion, is about 6 inches above the body surface, the entire motion taking approximately 5 seconds. The hand may then be relaxed, slightly so that the fingers slant slightly downwards, and the hand is returned to the starting position, at the crown chakra.

While performing the downward motion, visualize, with the intention that the *Angelic-Reiki Healing Angels* clear and cleans the auric field of your client; removing all impurities.

The practitioner hands will be activated by the *Angelic-Reiki Healing Angels* and act as a magnet which unfastens the harmful energies from the client's auric field. Apart from the client's body, these toxic energies lose their charge, and their ability to cling to the energy field of the client.

The toxins will dissolve, and become neutral energy, and have no further effect on the client. However, at this point the practitioner should ask that this neutral energy be turned into positive energy that the earth can use.

Using the motion detailed above, feel the energy in your hand and fingers, feel the field around your fingers expanding and growing strong, and visualize, intend and sense it attracting, pulling and clearing away the undesirable energies as you draw your hand outwards.

Repeat this motion as many times as necessary.

This will usually involve at least 3 hand-passings; however, it is possible to take up to eleven hand-passings to remove a highly toxic auric field.

Some practitioners like to "shake" the impurities off their hand, after the hand is fully drawn down the client's body. It is also recommended to have a basin (bowl) of warm salted water for the practitioner to place their hands in. The salted water will quickly neutralize and reground the practitioner, before performing the next drawing-out motion.

This treatment will be required at various points all over the body. The energies that the practitioner will clear are energies that have been stagnate and may appear to you the practitioner as muddied, thick, or discolored, energies that hinder the open flow of clear energy. These stagnant energies accumulate near the body surface, they are attached to the body and will extend a short distance into the body if not removed, causing an unbalance to the client.

Performing an *Angelic-Reiki Aura Clearing* will remove such blocks, for the area stagnant energy that is just below or above the body.

You will find that aura clearing will also be required over specific chakras, some quite more often than other. The 7th, 4th, and 2nd chakras are particularly vulnerable to these sorts of stagnant energies.

It is highly recommended to do an *Angelic-Reiki Chakra Balancing* after the aura clearing.

Remember: at the end of the **Aura Clearing Sessions** to use **Angelic-Reiki Energy Healing, Charged Holy Water™,** this seals the clearing process. 3 sprits one spritz at the Crown Chakra, the second should be spritzed over the trunk of the client, and the third spritz should be at the foot of the client.

.

To help keep the <u>Auric Field Clear</u> of negative debris it is recommended to use three spritzes of
Angelic-Reiki Energy Healing
Aura Clearing Holy Water ™
at the end of each day, or as needed.
Spray three sprites over the Crown Chakra.

Chapter 6

Soul-Cords and Event-Cords

Vs.

Spiritual Ribbons and Spiritual Ties

Soul-Cords and Event-Cords vs. Spiritual Ribbons

<u>What are Soul-Cords and Event-Cords</u>

Soul-Cords and Event-Cords are Spiritual Cords and Attachments we carry from people and events we have experience throughout our life. Yes, even *Events* in our lives can form a cord; attaching us to a particular time and space; these *Negative and Damaging Cords* must be severed for the *Human Being* to move forward into an existence of Health and Happiness.

A Soul-Cord is a spiritual energy attachment between two people; these cords may cause a person to repeat a behavioral pattern that is harmful to the spiritual development of the individual. Cords can drain personal energy, alter a person's thinking, manipulate their emotions, and affect the physical body, causing physical and psychological damage.

Event-Cords, just as *Soul Cords* are energy attachments, however, an Event-Cord attaches to the *Human Being* by a negative, harmful event that happens in their life.

Soul-Cord and Event-Cord Attachments are formations that if you could physically view would look like a nylon rope approximately 1/4 inch thick;

however as time passes the cord becomes stronger and thicker, some may grow to over an inch in thickness; and for this reason it is vital for the *Human Being* to remove these cords, as soon as they are identified.

Soul-Cord and Event-Cord can attach at any *Chakra*, except for the *Crown Chakra*. Keeping the *Chakras System* clear and balanced of these cords help to prevent energy loss and Cord attachments.

Spiritual Ties and Spiritual Ribbons

Spiritual Ties:
Spiritual Ties are not cords of attachment. However, relationships and events in our lives create these Spiritual Ties, just as they create Soul-Cords and Event-Cords.

Spiritual Ties bring positive energy, beauty, love, joy, inspiration, happiness, pleasure, and wonders into our physical and spiritual lives.

They are of the Light and do not bind, instead these Spiritual Ties wrap around us like Angelic Wings.

Spiritual Ribbons:

Spiritual Ribbons are the opposite of a *Soul-Cord or Event Cord. **Spiritual Ribbons cannot be removed.***

They are the ribbons that flow from the Heavens.

Spiritual Ribbons *attach to the Human Being* through the *Crown Chakra* and flow throughout the human body. For this reason it is vital to keep the **Crown Chakra** clean and balanced.

Spiritual Ribbons Are Divinely Sent Bringing Inspiration, Happiness, Wisdom, Gentleness, Love, Compassion, Good Physical Health and Good Psychological Health.

> **Note:** *The Human Being will never ever be confused between Spiritual Ties and Spiritual Ribbons, which are of the Light and Soul-Cords and Event-Cords, which are not!*

Chapter 7

Angelic-Reiki Cord Release
Releasing Soul-Cords and Event-Cords

Releasing Soul-Cords and Event-Cords

Note: Please remember we are Spiritual Healers, not Psychological Healers or Medical Doctors

The Human Being should always embrace life, and never, ever lose who they truly are. They should remain true.

"To Thy Own Self Be True"

By releasing Soul-Cords and Event-Cords, we stop inhaling the energy of the negative person or event. We release the energy that traps the Human Being in time and space. We also heal the Karma that goes along with these attachments.

We heal these Cord Releasings with *Angelic-Reiki Energy Healing.* This Healing Session will permanently heals and changes the Client's soul.

The *Client* as well as the person on the other end of the Soul-Cord will receive the *Angelic-Reiki Energy Healing.*

Releasing Soul-Cords and Event-Cords does not always mean ending a relationship. It means releasing the negative energy that repeat on an endless loop.

Releasing Soul-Cords and Event-Cords will clear away the negative cords that should have not been attached.

Releasing Soul-Cords and Event-Cords will heal any energy that remains from the attachment.

Releasing Soul-Cords and Event-Cords will give the Client a feeling of being lighter or more grounded, improving their Spiritual and Physical Energy, and also improving their emotional and physical health.

Angelic-Reiki Energy Healing Sessions are permanent changes to the Soul.

Remember: to use **Angelic-Reiki Energy Healing, Charged Holy Water™,** at the beginning of each Angelic-Reiki Energy Cord Release.

Spray three spritzes at the Crown Chakra of the client before beginning the Angelic-Reiki Energy Healing Soul-Cord and Event-Cord Release.

Angelic-Reiki Energy Healing
Soul-Cords and Event-Cords Procedure

We work with the *Angelic-Reiki Healing Angels*.
Begin by calling on **The *Archangel Raphael;*** now
ask for the *Angels of Angelic- Reiki* to join you, to
become one with you; that you both may become
one.

First you begin with this Prayer of Protection.

Prayer for Spiritual Protection
Guardian Angels of the Heavenly Realm,
Circle round protection bound
Stand tall guarding our gates
Ever keeping safe our fate
In all Realms in all Space
In all Times
Sealed
With Grace

Cover yourself and your client with Angelic-
Reiki White Light. You may want to light a
white candle at this time to represent this angelic
protective energy.

1. Both you and your client should hold the intention that all Soul-Cords and Event-Cords will be released and replaced with positive Angelic-Reiki Energy.

2. Then release any Soul-Cords and Event-Cords that the client has sent out, ask that they be returned and replaced with Angelic Energy.

3. At this time the Practitioner will pass their hands over the client, starting at their Crown Chakra (the client may be sitting or standing during this procedure.)

4. The practitioner hand should be approximately six inches away from the client's body.

5. Both the practitioner and the client should visualize the cord gently being released as the practitioner slowly glides their hands down the outline of the client's torso.

6. The practitioner should pass their hand one in the front of the client, and the other at the back, slowly moving them down the client's torso, once they reach the Root/Base Chakra the practitioner should fan their hand outward away for the client and shake the energy of the cords off.

7. The practitioner should now return to the Crown Chakra and glide their hands slowly down the sides of the client, once more when reaching the Root/Base Chakra, fan their hands out and shake the energy off.

8. Some clients who are involved in a negative relationship may feel a popping off of these cords. This will cause the client to view their relationship in the correct light, and change the relationship, by changing themselves; suddenly they will have a completely different outlook on the relationship.

9. Also during the releasing of these cords any and all cords from past lives will be released, along with the Karma that accompanied them.

10. When completed please offer your client some water to drink, it will help ground them. They may need to sit for a while; this is a good time to offer some spiritual counseling.

Releasing Soul-Cords and Event-Cords is vital for the Human Being's healing and spiritual growth.

<u>**Remember**</u>**:** at the end of the healing sessions to use **Angelic-Reiki Energy Healing, Charged Holy Water™,** this seals the healing process. 3 sprits one spritz at the Crown Chakra, the second should be spritzed over the trunk of the client, and the third spritz should be at the foot of the client.

<u>**Also recommend:**</u>; for the client to continue the uses of **Angelic-Reiki Energy Healing, Charged Holy Water™,** for 9 days after the initial Healing Procedure. This enhances the gentleness of the healing process.

<u>**Remember**</u> the practitioner should have a small basin of water places in their Healing Room and a clean hand towel. In the basin should be warm water and a table spoon of Angelic-Reiki Energy Healing, Blessed Energy Balancing Salts™ mixed in it.

After each Angelic-Reiki Energy Healing, Procedure the practitioner should rinse and dry their hand to neutralize the energy that they have used during the healing session.

Chapter 9

Angelic-Reiki Healing
Meditation

Angelic-Reiki Healing Angels

Healing Meditation

You can work with the *Angelic-Reiki Healing Angels* and *Archangel Raphael* using meditation.

This Meditation may be used for your personal healing and also for your Clients.

To prepare Invoke the *Angelic-Reiki Healing Angels* and *Archangel Raphael,* to please help you open to their *Healing Energy* and support you through the healing process.

Sit comfortably where you will not be disturbed. Begin by grounding and centering yourself. Close your eyes and imagining roots growing from your feet into the Earth.

Follow this simple breathing exercise to relax your physical body: breathe in through your nose, hold it for several seconds, and release it very slowly through your mouth.

Continue breathing this way throughout the meditation.

Ask *The Divine Creator* to send down a beam of protective white light. Envision a beam of light coming down from the Heavens. Watch it surround you and your client, placing you both in a protective sphere.

This Sphere of White Light is protecting you and your client in all time, all realms, and all space.

Call to Angelic-Reiki Healing Angels and Archangel Raphael, asking. "Angels of Healing please come to me now and assist me in this healing." "Spirit Guides and Guardian Angels, please join The Angelic-Reiki Angels in this/my healing session."

In your mind's eye, picture The Angelic-Reiki Angels standing over you and your client. See the healing energy in the form of green light flowing down into your body and or the body of your client. It is flowing through the Crown Chakra. Relax and feel this *Divine Healing Energy.*

Both you and your client will feel the *Angelic-Reiki Healing Energy* as warmth or tingling running through their body.

Let this energy flow through you for a while, opening you and your client to this *Divine Healing Energy* and preparing you on all levels for the healing.

This initial step may last for several minutes, until you feel that it is time to move on to the next step.

Now change your focus to specific parts of the body. Picture the green light of healing energy flowing through the *Angelic-Reiki Healing Angels* and *Archangel Raphael*, to the injury or area of illness.

When you are finished, thank the *Angelic-Reiki Healing Angels* and *Archangel Raphael*, for protecting you from all negative thoughts and feelings that manifest into health problems. Also thank your Spirit Guides and Angels for assisting in this healing.

Focus once more on grounding and centering yourself.

Now open your eyes.

The *Angelic-Reiki Healing Angels* and *Archangel Raphael* along with *Divine Intervention* are what you are healed by.

It does not matter if you are good at visualization.

You may repeat this meditation whenever you feel it is necessary.

This meditation works with injuries and illnesses.

Chapter 10

Wrapping Up
Level 1

You have just completed your first level to becoming an Ordained Angelic-Reiki Energy Healing Master.

Please remember that the Angelic Chakra Alignment will be a 40-day process. It is highly recommended that you keep a journal of your experiences during this adjustment period.

You will open up to a much higher frequency than you have ever been accustomed to, and you will be bestowed with many Spiritual Gifts.

My blessings are with you as you begin this Noble and Honorable Journey into…

…The Art of Angelic-Reiki Energy Healing™

May You Be Wrapped In Angelic Wings!

My Wish for You

As Always...

May The Powers That Be

Bless You Indeed

With health, wealth

And prosperity

With

Wisdom to share

And

Courage to lead

May They guard your gate

Always keeping safe

Your fate.

Rev. Debbie Michaels

Notes

Notes

Notes

Notes

Notes

Notes

Notes

Notes